Proven, Natural Solutions for Depression, Osteoarthritis and Liver Health

with iSO ACTIVE High Isomer SAMe

Sherry Torkos, B.Sc. Phm.

This book is intended for educational and informational purposes only. Please see a qualified medical professional if you have questions about your health.

Library and Archives Canada Cataloguing in Publication

Torkos, Sherry
Proven natural solutions for depression, osteoarthritis and liver health / Sherry Torkos.

ISBN 0-470-83612-1

1. Depression, Mental—Alternative treatment. 2. Osteoarthritis—Alternative treatment. 3. Liver—Diseases—Alternative treatment. 4. Naturopathy. I. Title.

RZ440.T67 2004 615.5'55 C2004-904914-3

Production Credit

Cover design: Adrian So R.G.D.
Interior text design: Natalia Burobina
Printer: Tri-Graphic Printing Ltd.

Printed in Canada

10 9 8 7 6 5 4 3 2 1

Contents

CONTENTS

Introduction 1
Isoactive SAMe: Nature's Newest Superstar 2
Understanding How SAMe Works 3
Dealing with Depression 6
SAMe and Depression 9
Supporting Research on Depression 10
Using SAMe for Depression 13
Patient Case 1: Depression 14
Patient Case 2: Depression 15
An Expert's Perspective 16
Osteoarthritis 21
Alleviating Osteoarthritis 24
The Perils of Prescription Drugs for Osteoarthritis 24
SAMe and Osteoarthritis 27
Supporting Research on Osteoarthritis 27
Patient Case 3: Osteoarthritis 30
Patient Case 4: Osteoarthritis 31
Fibromyalgia/Chronic Fatigue Syndrome 33
Supporting Research on Fibromyalgia 35
Liver Disorders 37
Supporting Research on Liver Disorders 37
Anti-aging 40
New Areas of Research 42
Supplementing with SAMe 43
Adverse Reactions 44
Interactions 44
Dosage Guidelines and Storage 44
Buyer Be Wise 45
Natural Isoactive versus Synthetic SAMe 46
Conclusion 47
References 48

Introduction

INTRODUCTION

The nutritional supplement industry has become a multibillion dollar business. The use of vitamins, minerals, herbs, and other natural supplements continues to rise in popularity as mounting research supports the benefits of these natural products for improving health and wellness.

There is another reason for the growing interest in natural medicine—frustration with conventional medicine, which focuses on the use of drugs and surgery. While these Western approaches to disease can offer life-saving treatments for certain conditions, they do little to address chronic diseases, and are associated with many side effects and health risks. Chronic diseases such as heart disease, diabetes, cancer, arthritis, and depression continue to plague our society and are leading causes of death, disability, and financial burden.

Working as a pharmacist for over twelve years, I have seen first hand the limitations of prescription drug use—side effects that can often be worse than the condition for which the drug was prescribed, numerous drug interactions, and escalating costs. I have seen the sick get sicker when they are reliant solely on prescription drugs for their health. The majority of drugs that we have today address the symptoms of disease, offering a bandage-type approach, rather than addressing the underlying cause.

I find that consumers today are looking for more—they want safer, more cost-effective *natural* alternatives, such as those provided by the field of holistic or complementary medicine.

Isoactive SAMe

ISOACTIVE SAMe: NATURE'S NEWEST SUPERSTAR

One of the greatest discoveries in complementary medicine is a naturally occurring substance called SAMe (pronounced "Sammy"). *Newsweek* magazine was the first to point a national spotlight on SAMe, the natural health industry's newest superstar. Articles have also appeared in *Time, USA Today,* and the *Globe and Mail.* Soon after, "ABC Nightly News" and "Dateline" featured the benefits of SAMe, making it one of the most talked about natural substances to hit the mass market since St. John's wort. Oddly enough, just like St. John's wort, SAMe's claim to fame is connected with depression. I'll delve into that issue a little later, but first, what is this new natural sensation?

SAMe is an abbreviation for S-adenosyl-methionine. It is a substance made in the human body when the amino acid methionine (which is found in protein-rich foods such as fish, meat, and dairy products) combines with adenosine triphosphate (ATP). SAMe was first identified in Italy almost fifty years ago and has been popular in Europe ever since. The excitement surrounding SAMe and the knowledge of its numerous health benefits has spread to North America and other areas of the world, making it an international success.

SAMe is vital to the health and development of many tissues and organs in the human body. It is involved in more than forty biochemical reactions and specific processes, such as detoxification, brain function, and joint health. With the help of folic acid and vitamin B12, SAMe makes a positive contribution to almost every bodily function. It truly is a dynamic and exciting substance.

While SAMe is produced in the body, there are a number of conditions that can create a deficiency of this nutrient. An inadequate intake of methionine, vitamin B12, or folic acid can result in decreased SAMe synthesis. The elderly and those suffering from osteoarthritis, depression, and various liver disorders are known to have lower levels of SAMe. Interestingly, supplementing with SAMe has been found to benefit these conditions.

Understanding How

UNDERSTANDING HOW SAMe WORKS

Researchers consider SAMe to be one of the most active methyl donors in the human body. A methyl donor is a molecule that gives up a methyl group (a four-atom cluster consisting of one carbon unit and three hydrogen molecules) to another molecule, so that molecule can carry out its prescribed duties. This ongoing process is known as methylation and takes place in the human body about a billion times per second.

Methylation regulates, controls, and influences everything from gene expression to hormone activity to neurotransmitter development. As a valuable methyl donor, SAMe is involved in the production of nucleic acids (DNA, RNA), proteins, certain vitamins, neurotransmitters, antioxidants, hormones, and phospholipids. SAMe is also involved in the biosynthesis of many sulfur-containing compounds, including the antioxidant glutathione, the amino acids taurine and cysteine, and the sulfur-containing components of connective tissue. It is also part of the detoxification process.

As you can imagine, this process of methylation is absolutely critical to life. "Without methylation, there could be no life as we know it," explains biochemist Craig Cooney, author of *Methyl Magic: Maximum Health through Methylation* (Kansas City: Andrews McMeel Publishing, 1999). That's one reason SAMe is getting so much attention.

SAMe is created when methionine combines with adenosine triphosphate (ATP), a key energy source for cells.

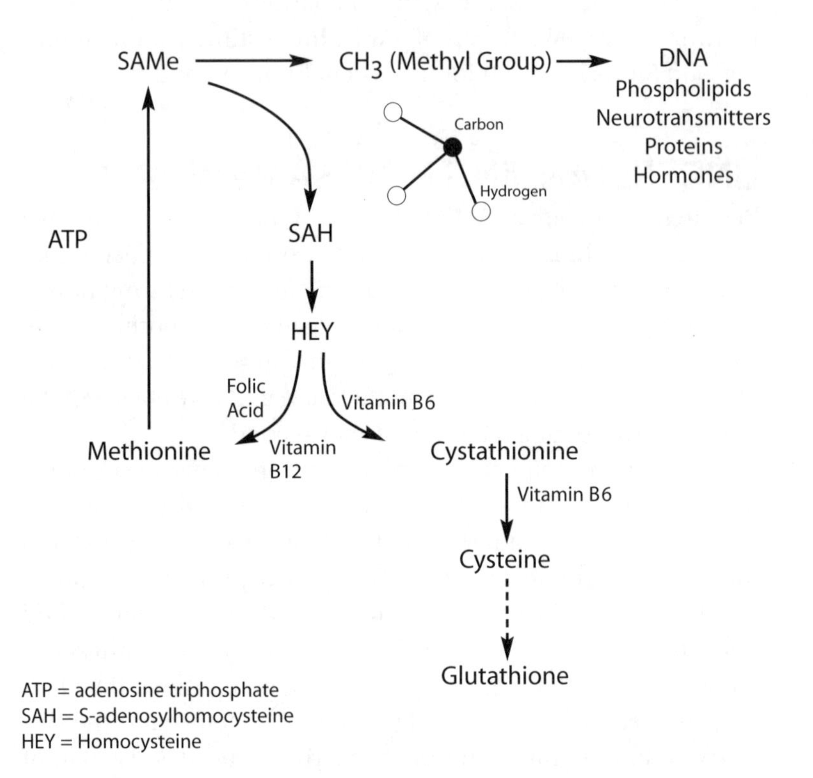

Perhaps the most significant contribution occurs when SAMe gives up its methyl group to another molecule. SAMe then turns into homocysteine, which can become toxic if there is not enough folic acid and vitamin B12 available. These two important vitamins combine with homocysteine to convert it into glutathione, a valuable antioxidant. For this reason, it is important to take folic acid and vitamin B12 along with SAMe.

Because SAMe functions on a cellular level and is involved in several different vital processes within the body, its therapeutic benefits are far-reaching and varied. This causes some scientists to lift a suspicious eyebrow at the idea of a "cure-all." While SAMe is certainly not a cure-all, solid scientific research is available in four key areas: (1) depression, (2) osteoarthritis, (3) fibromyalgia, and (4) liver disorders.

Most importantly, the benefits of SAMe have been backed by numerous clinical studies. In the natural products industry, where many products offer false promises, SAMe is a rare and truly unique product—a superstar.

For more than twenty years, European physicians have been using SAMe as an approved prescription drug to treat both depression and osteoarthritis. SAMe is available without a prescription as a dietary supplement in the United States and, recently, in Canada. In Canada, SAMe was available without a prescription as a dietary supplement until 2002, when the government decided to suspend over-the-counter sales until a review of the research could be evaluated. There was speculation in the natural products industry that SAMe's removal from the market may have been prompted by the pharmaceutical industry. At the time this occurred, it had been getting a great deal of attention in the media as a safer alternative to prescription antidepressants. When Health Canada introduced the new regulations for dietary supplements in 2004, SAMe became available again, as its safety and efficacy was well-documented.

While SAMe should not be considered a "magic bullet," the growing scientific evidence is impressive. As you read through this booklet, I will be referring to the benefits of supplementing with SAMe. SAMe supplements exist in both natural and synthetic (generic) forms. For many reasons, which are outlined in the "Buyer Be Wise" section of this booklet, the natural form of SAMe is preferred and recommended. The natural form is sold under the name ISOACTIVE High Isomer SAMe. This is what you should look for on a label when choosing a SAMe supplement.

Let's begin by evaluating the scientific research on SAMe and depression. But first, a word of caution. *Keep in mind that this booklet is intended for educational purposes. If you have a specific health condition you are concerned about, or would like to alter medications you are presently taking, please see a qualified health care professional.*

DEALING WITH DEPRESSION

Dealing with Depression

Anxiety and depression are the most common psychiatric ailment in Western society. In fact, depression affects more than 17 million people every year in the United States. Approximately one in eight Americans—25 percent of all women and 12 percent of all men—are diagnosed with serious depression at some point in their lives.

Approximately 1.4 million people in Canada are afflicted at any given time. Over $3 billion is spent on the direct medical costs associated with this disease. Depression is the second leading cause of long-term disability among workers, number one among white-collar workers, and the fourth leading cause of global burden of disease; it is projected to be the second leading cause by 2020.

According to the American Psychiatric Association's *Diagnostic Manual of Mental Disorders,* serious clinical depression has the following symptoms:

- poor appetite and significant weight loss, or increased appetite and significant weight gain
- insomnia or increased sleep
- agitation or sluggishness in movement and thought
- loss of interest or pleasure in usual activities, or decrease in sexual drive

- fatigue or loss of energy
- feelings of worthlessness, self-reproach, or excessive or inappropriate guilt
- diminished ability to think or concentrate, or indecisiveness
- recurrent thoughts of death or suicide, or suicide attempts

An individual is considered depressed if he or she exhibits four or more of the above symptoms nearly every day for at least two weeks.

[**NOTE:** *If you or someone you know is seriously depressed, it is imperative to consult a qualified health care professional without delay. Self-treatment is not recommended.]*

There are many known causes of depression: environmental (exposure to chemicals that disrupt brain chemistry), nutritional (deficiency of certain vitamins), situational (stress), and physiological (imbalance of neurotransmitters). Whenever possible, it is important that the underlying cause be determined so that an appropriate treatment can be initiated. For example, cases of depression have been linked to chemical exposure, such as inhalation of fumes given off by new carpet or paints, ingestion of chemicals in food (dyes, preservatives, pesticides), or skin contact with chemicals found in cosmetics, lotions, or other topical products. In these cases, eliminating exposure to the toxin can often resolve the problem, although it may take some time. Often, however, it is difficult to determine the underlying cause and an individual may need to consult a doctor trained in environmental or functional medicine.

Conventional treatment of depression includes the use of prescription drugs and psychiatric counseling. Antidepressant drugs are divided into two major categories: tricyclic drugs and newer selective serotonin re-uptake inhibitors (SSRIs). Tricyclic antidepressants include amitriptyline, clomipramine, imipramine, nortriptyline, desipramine, and doxepin. The SSRIs include fluoxetine, fluvoxamine, citalopram, paroxetine, and sertraline. While these drugs have helped many individuals, some professionals believe they are being prescribed too frequently and that safer alternatives should be explored.

The main concern with antidepressant drugs is their high incidence of side effects, drug interactions, and variable response. In fact, some estimates show that one-third of individuals taking these drugs will not be helped or are unable to tolerate the side effects. Side effects include, but are not limited to:

- nausea and/or loss of appetite
- headaches
- anxiety and nervousness
- insomnia or drowsiness
- diarrhea
- sweating and tremors
- loss of libido and reduced sex drive
- agitation

It seems as though some patients taking antidepressive medications have been paying a high price for their relief in terms of side effects and cost. On average, a prescription for a new-generation antidepressant costs $50–$60 a month in Canada and $80–$120 in the United States. Perhaps this is why natural substances such as St. John's wort and SAMe receive so much attention.

Clinical studies have shown that SAMe is not only effective, but also free of serious side effects. SAMe is more costly than the average nutritional supplement, but it is much less expensive than a prescription. On the other hand, health insurance benefits don't usually pay for SAMe. This is starting to change, however, as health insurance providers see the value in providing coverage for supplements—fewer side effects—which can translate into cost savings in the long term. In fact, in my pharmacy practice, there are several cases where individuals received coverage for natural products through their health insurance plan when the product was prescribed by a doctor and accompanied by a letter indicating the reason for prescribing the natural product (such as SAMe) instead of a drug. Hopefully in the future our health care system will start to acknowledge the value of natural products and provide coverage, and thus greater access, to these items.

SAMe and Depression

Most of the initial research on the benefits of SAMe focused on depression. It was found that individuals diagnosed with depression had low plasma levels of SAMe. This makes sense when you consider the importance of methylation to regulating brain function and mood.

SAMe is essential for the manufacture of brain neurotransmitters (chemical messengers) such as dopamine, norepinephrine, epinephrine, and serotonin. Low levels of these neurotransmitters are associated with depression. SAMe supports the binding of these neurotransmitters to their receptor sites, thus enhancing their activity. It may also accelerate the production, uptake, and re-release of the main mood regulator, serotonin. By methylating certain phospholipids (fatty molecules that are crucial to the health of cell membranes), such as phosphatidylcholine and phosphatidylserine, in the cell membranes, SAMe also enhances cell membrane fluidity and improves cellular communication between neurons. Together, all of these actions alleviate depression.

Supporting Research on Depression

In October 2002, the U.S. Department of Health and Human Services, Agency for Healthcare Research and Quality (AHRQ) released an evidence report on the use of SAMe for the treatment of depression, osteoarthritis, and liver disease. AHRQ is a U.S. federal agency charged with supporting research designed to improve the quality of health care, reduce its cost, address patient safety and medical errors, and broaden access to essential services.

The investigators involved in this project identified 102 relevant studies that included SAMe for the treatment of depression, osteoarthritis, or liver disease. With respect to depression, forty-seven studies were reviewed and twenty-eight met the criteria to be included in the meta-analysis (review) of SAMe for depression. In these twenty-eight studies the efficacy of SAMe in reducing the symptoms of depression was compared to either a placebo or a conventional antidepressant. The researchers concluded that "Compared to placebo, treatment with SAMe was associated with an improvement of approximately 6 points in the score of the Hamilton Rating Scale for Depression. [This scale is commonly used to gauge response to treatment.] This degree of improvement is statistically and clinically significant and is equivalent to a partial response to treatment." It was also stated that "Compared to treatment with conventional therapy, SAMe was not associated with a statistically significant difference in outcomes." Simply put, SAMe was found to be more effective than a placebo and just as effective as conventional antidepressants in improving the symptoms of depression.

One limitation of this review is that it was not designed to compare tolerability (side effects) or cost effectiveness of SAMe versus conventional antidepressants. SAMe is certainly more cost effective than the new-generation antidepressants (SSRIs) yet more expensive than the older antidepressants (tricyclics). With respect to side effects, many individual studies have compared SAMe to the antidepressant drugs and SAMe comes out a winner—it has fewer side effects and is much better tolerated. SAMe has not been found to cause any significant side effects. In fact, while some antidepressants cause liver damage, SAMe has actually been shown in numerous studies to protect the liver—another benefit of this superstar.

In another meta-analysis published in Denmark (Bell KM, et al, 1994), researchers concluded that SAMe was more effective than a placebo, just as effective as prescribed tricyclic medications, and very safe. They called SAMe a "potentially important treatment for depression."

Here are some highlights of a few recent studies conducted on SAMe for depression:

- *University La Sapienza, Rome (2002):* This multicenter study compared the effects of intramuscularly (i.m.) administered SAMe to imipramine (IMI) in 293 patients with major depression over four weeks. The authors concluded "400 mg/d i.m. SAMe to be comparable to 150 mg/d oral IMI in terms of antidepressive efficacy, but significantly better tolerated."
- *Beth Israel Medical Center-Albert Einstein College of Medicine, New York (2000):* This study examined the effects of SAMe on thirteen depressed patients with Parkinson's disease. All the patients had been previously treated with other antidepressant agents and had no significant benefit or had intolerable side effects. SAMe was administered in doses of 800–3600 mg per day for ten weeks. Eleven patients completed the study, and ten had at least a 50 percent improvement on the seventeen-point Hamilton Depression Scale (HDS). One patient did not improve and two patients dropped out because of increased anxiety. Side effects were mild and transient. Although this study was small, the authors concluded

that "SAMe is well tolerated and may be a safe and effective alternative to the antidepressant agents currently used in patients with Parkinson's disease."

- *Massachusetts General Hospital, Boston (1995):* This study evaluated the ability of SAMe to reduce the delay in antidepressant response, since SAMe appears to have a rapid onset of effect in the treatment of depression. In this open, multicenter study, 195 patients were given 400 mg of SAMe, administered by injection, for fifteen days. It was concluded that "Depressive symptoms remitted after both 7 and 15 days of treatment with SAMe, and no serious adverse events were reported."
- *University of California-Irvine Medical Center, Irvine (1994):* Following a four-week study of twenty-six patients, researchers concluded that "The significant correlation between plasma SAMe levels and the degree of clinical improvement in depressed patients regardless of type of treatment suggests that SAMe may play an important role in regulating mood."
- *University La Sapienza School of Medicine, Rome (1993):* A group of eighty postmenopausal women between the ages of forty-five and fifty-nine, diagnosed with major depressive disorder, participated in this thirty-day, double-blind, placebo-controlled trial. The women were between six and thirty-six months following either natural menopause or hysterectomy. They underwent one week of single-blind placebo washout, followed by thirty days of double-blind treatment with either 1600 mg of SAMe per day or a placebo. The researchers concluded that "There was a significantly greater improvement in depressive symptoms . . . observed in the patients treated with SAMe compared to the placebo group."

- *Mexican Institute of Psychiatry, Mexico City (1992):* This double-blind clinical trial evaluated the efficacy of SAMe in speeding the onset of action of imipramine, a tricyclic antidepressant. Forty patients with moderate to severe depression received either 200 mg per day of SAMe intramuscularly with 150 mg per day of imipramine, or a placebo with imipramine. Researchers found that the depressive symptoms decreased earlier in the patients receiving SAMe and imipramine, than in those receiving a placebo and imipramine.

Using SAMe for Depression

Most studies using SAMe for depression used dosages of 400–1600 mg daily. It would be best to start with 400 mg and gradually increase the dosage as needed. While SAMe works more quickly than conventional antidepressants, allow one to two weeks for optimal effect. Again, if you are on a prescription medication for depression, do not discontinue it without proper medical supervision.

Based on the results from both human and animal studies, SAMe appears to be quite safe. As with conventionally prescribed antidepressants, SAMe should not be used to treat bipolar disorder (i.e., manic-depression), as it can worsen the manic symptoms.

Often individuals are worried about adverse interactions, which can occur when certain pharmaceutical and/or natural compounds are combined. Presently, no adverse interactions are documented in the scientific literature for SAMe. European historical use, as well as clinical research, indicates that SAMe is safe even at higher dosages, such as greater than 1200 mg daily. Although it has not been documented in the scientific literature, some people report a reduced appetite when taking SAMe. Some individuals have also reported nausea and gastrointestinal upset at higher dosages (1600 mg or more). If this occurs, reduce the dosage or take SAMe with a small piece of bread or a cracker. Typically, SAMe should be taken on an empty stomach for optimal absorption. For more information about what to look for when purchasing SAMe, refer to the "Buyer Be Wise" section beginning on page 45.

Patient Case 1: Depression

DESCRIPTION

Julie was a forty-six-year-old woman who was diagnosed with depression seven years ago. Her symptoms included fatigue, insomnia, weight gain, lack of motivation, feelings of worthlessness, and reduced libido. Julie commented that she "had no desire to live" and was "tired of feeling depressed."

PREVIOUS TREATMENT

Previous medications included conventionally prescribed tricyclics and SSRIs. Many of the medications worked initially, but the benefits tapered off over time and she was unable to tolerate the side effects. She had tried St. John's wort, but developed a rash and had to discontinue it.

RECOMMENDATIONS

I recommended that Julie consider trying SAMe. She discussed it with her physician, who was somewhat familiar with the product and agreed that she should give it a try since many of the conventional products had not worked for her. She began taking 400 mg daily. After one week, she increased her dosage to 400 mg twice daily.

FOLLOW-UP

After three weeks, Julie reported that she noticed a marked improvement in her mood, emotional state, and well-being. She had more energy and reported that, overall, she felt better.

Patient Case 2: Depression

DESCRIPTION

John, fifty-two, was diagnosed with moderate depression following the loss of his job and the resulting financial stress that his family experienced. His symptoms included fatigue, feelings of sadness, doom and gloom, and loss of appetite.

PREVIOUS TREATMENT

John had tried various medications and had gone to several psychiatrists over the past few years as he tried to find a treatment that would make him feel better. Even though he had found another job and had less financial stress, the depression continued and he struggled with unpleasant side effects with every drug he tried. He did find some relief with an SSRI, but the sexual side effects that he experienced were upsetting and creating a strain on his marriage, so he stopped taking it. While his doctor encouraged him to continue, John commented that "the treatment was almost as bad as the disease" and that the side effects were "depressing."

RECOMMENDATIONS

When John came to see me, I suggested that he talk to his doctor about SAMe. Since he had tried most of the newest drugs and was unable to tolerate their side effects, I thought that SAMe was worth a try. SAMe also has a quicker onset of action. John talked with his doctor, who was not familiar with SAMe. I supplied the doctor with a review of the clinical research on SAMe and recommendations for use. He was impressed with the information and agreed to give it a try with John. We agreed to start him on 400 mg daily and increase it if needed after the second week.

FOLLOW-UP

After only two weeks of using SAMe, John reported that his mood and energy level had improved. He was sleeping better at night and had more energy during the day. After four weeks, John said that he felt better than he had in years. He could not believe that there were no side effects with this product because with all the drugs that he had tried in the past, the side effects would become pronounced and intolerable within the first month of use. SAMe was continued at 400 mg daily and John followed up with his doctor every six months thereafter.

An Expert's Perspective

Dr. Richard Brown, Columbia University psychiatrist and co-author of *Stop Depression Now* (New York: Putnam, 1999), commented that SAMe is "the best antidepressant I've ever prescribed." To get further insight into the topic of SAMe and depression, my colleague, Karolyn Gazella, interviewed Dr. Brown.

Q. *How did you get started using SAMe?*

A. I had read a good deal about it, including several studies conducted by Teodoro Bottiglieri, Ph.D. (co-author of *Stop Depression Now*). I was impressed by the research and began using SAMe on my patients a few years ago. I started giving SAMe to patients who hadn't responded to antidepressants, either at all or only partially, and also to patients who had been unable to tolerate antidepressant treatment because of side effects. And then I saw that SAMe not only worked as often as standard antidepressants, but people seemed to feel much better physically while taking it. They didn't feel medicated at all, as they did with standard prescription antidepressants. They would often tell me about ways in which they physically felt better after weeks or months of treatment.

Q. *Do you recommend SAMe as a first-line treatment for mild, moderate, and severe depression?*

A. It is important to understand that every individual is different. Also, the way physicians and patients classify their degree of depression can be somewhat subjective. Overall, however, I find SAMe to be helpful across the board for varying degrees of depression. Certainly, it is a good treatment choice for mild depression, including seasonal depression. Although there are no studies on seasonal depression at this point, I have had good clinical results. I also think it is very good for moderate depression and sometimes severe depression. In cases of severe depression, it may have to be combined with other prescriptions.

Q. *How does SAMe compare to St. John's wort, the herbal extract that received national media attention two years ago for its ability to alleviate symptoms of mild to moderate depression?*

A. I use St. John's wort a lot and I was very glad that it became available for over-the-counter use. I think both SAMe and St. John's wort serve a valuable purpose. A large number of people suffer from mild depression. They will not go for help because their symptoms are not severe enough or they don't want to take standard prescription antidepressants because they've heard about the side effects.

I have seen a lot of people helped by St. John's wort. It is not a placebo. St. John's wort, however, is more of a mild antidepressant. There have only been twenty-five studies with St. John's wort, with only the last two involving severe depression. In these last two studies, a higher dose of St. John's wort was used to get results—about double what the previous studies had used. Unfortunately, most consumers who take St. John's wort take the lower dose. And those people taking the higher dose experience more side effects. In my clinical practice, I have seen the same side effects as with prescription SSRIs in patients taking the higher dosages of St. John's wort. These symptoms include sexual dysfunction, insomnia, jaw clenching, nausea, and mild to severe sun sensitivity and rash.

SAMe has far fewer side effects, and those are typically temporary. In addition, SAMe works much faster. You don't see great benefits from St. John's wort in many cases for a few months. A lot of patients experiencing depression need pretty immediate improvement. To me, that's one of the great benefits of taking SAMe. A lot of patients feel better in a very short time. This is also important for compliance. Patients will continue taking a medication if it makes them feel better quicker.

To me, SAMe is better than St. John's wort. It seems to work more often and has more advantages in terms of overall physical well-being.

Q. *What has impressed you the most about SAMe?*

A. I'd say it's the feeling of well-being that people have while on it and how good they feel about taking it. It still amazes me how often my patients who are taking SAMe tell other people about it because they want them to get the same benefit. You don't see this type of testimonial with prescription antidepressants. It is impressive that it has hardly any significant side effects, works faster for many people, and generates important antioxidants that can do other good things in the body. That doesn't mean that it is perfect for everyone or that it cures everything. However, it is a very promising natural substance.

Q. *Can you comment about some of the other conditions SAMe has been studied for, specifically arthritis, fibromyalgia, and liver disorders?*

A. The data on arthritis are very clear and the results have been dramatic. There are twenty studies, with some comparing SAMe to nonsteroidal anti-inflammatory drugs (NSAIDs). In the case of arthritis, SAMe works extremely well and is a whole lot more tolerable than conventional treatments.

The studies on liver disorders have also been promising. This is a very important area that needs to be explored further.

There are six studies on fibromyalgia using SAMe treatment. I believe there is no other substance that has been studied this well for this condition. I've seen a lot of fibromyalgia patients over the years because it was, and still is by some medical doctors, thought to be a psychiatric disorder. Years ago, I was getting a lot of referrals of patients diagnosed with fibromyalgia. I quickly learned that these patients weren't like any depressed or psychiatric patient I've ever seen. They did not react to psychotropic medications like people who were depressed or anxious. They actually had bad reactions to the medications. I began trying to look for other things that may help them. SAMe is one of the few things that has actually been studied for this condition. Patients get results and the medication is so much better tolerated with few, if any, side effects. SAMe is not a cure for fibromyalgia, but I think it is quite helpful, in many cases, for relieving symptoms. Research should continue in this area.

Q. *What is the most exciting area of future research for SAMe?*

A. I am focusing on the areas of dementia and neurological disorders. I think SAMe can be helpful with depression secondary to neurological and medical conditions. This is the most important research that I am involved with right now.

One of my goals in writing the book [*Stop Depression Now*] was that I'd hoped it would restimulate research with SAMe here in the United States. The fact is, that is happening even faster than I had imagined.

Q. *How can individuals be sure that they are purchasing a quality product?*

A. They must purchase an enteric-coated, stabilized form of SAMe from a manufacturer with a long history and good reputation.

Q. *What is the most important information you would like to convey regarding SAMe and depression?*

A. SAMe is not a miracle cure—no pill is—but it does have a lot of advantages. It is easy to take and it works fast. However, individuals must also look at other things they can do. They must change their diet, lifestyle, and attitude. They need to reduce stress and find ways to manage their depression for the long run. I think the dietary link has really been overlooked by doctors. How are people's nerves going to respond to medicine if the nerves aren't getting proper nutrition? Nutrients are extremely important to the health of the nervous system. There is more research going on in this area, but even more needs to be done. I consider the dietary link to be crucial. The most successful antidepression program must be comprehensive.

[**NOTE:** For more information about a comprehensive treatment plan for depression, refer to Dr. Brown's book, *Stop Depression Now.*]

To review, here are the key benefits SAMe provides in the treatment of depression:

- It appears to be safer than commonly prescribed antidepressant medications, and has fewer side effects and drug interactions.

- It works fast. While other antidepressants (tricyclics, SSRIs, and St. John's wort) may take four to six weeks to work, SAMe users often experience relief within days.
- It has been shown to be just as effective as conventionally prescribed antidepressants.
- It is more affordable than conventional antidepressants.
- It is effective at reasonable dosages (400–1600 mg daily).

OSTEOARTHRITIS

Osteoarthritis

Osteoarthritis, also known as degenerative joint disease, is one of the most common types of arthritis. It is characterized by the breakdown of cartilage in the joint. Cartilage is normally present between the bones of a joint to provide cushioning. When the cartilage wears down, it causes bone to rub against bone, leading to pain and loss of movement.

According to the Osteoarthritis Foundation, this condition affects an estimated 20.7 million Americans, mostly after age forty-five. The pain, suffering, and financial burden caused by this condition are significant. Overall, musculoskeletal conditions, including osteoarthritis, cost the U.S. economy nearly $86.2 billion per year in direct expenses and lost wages and production. This is the second most common diagnosis—after chronic heart disease—that calls for Social Security disability payments due to long-term absence from work.

According to the 2000 Canadian Community Health Survey (CCHS), arthritis and other rheumatic conditions affected nearly 4 million Canadians aged fifteen and older (approximately one in six people), and is a leading cause of disability.

Compared to people with other chronic conditions, those with arthritis experienced more pain, activity restrictions, and long-term disability; were more likely to need help with daily activities; reported worse self-rated health and more disrupted sleep and depression; and reported more frequent contact with health care professionals in the previous year.

Osteoarthritis commonly affects middle-aged and older people, and it can range from very mild to very severe. It primarily affects wrists and weight-bearing joints such as knees, hips, feet, and the back, but may also be found in the neck, big toes, and fingers. It affects women more than men and virtually everyone over the age of seventy-five has some degree of osteoarthritis.

Stephen Katz, M.D., Ph.D., director of the National Institute of Arthritis and Musculoskeletal and Skin Diseases, states: "Arthritis is a leading cause of disability. With the aging population, it will increasingly burden individuals, as well as the economy." Additionally, researchers believe that as we age, the body's ability to repair joint cartilage decreases, and joint erosion increases.

While one's risk of developing osteoarthritis increases with age, this condition is not an inevitable part of aging. Genetics is known to be a factor: having a positive family history (e.i., having a parent or grandparent with the condition) increases your risk. Some individuals are born with defective cartilage or with slight defects in the way that joints fit together. As the person ages, these defects may cause the cartilage to break down in the joint, leading to inflammation, the release of certain enzymes, and then further cartilage damage.

Other risk factors include nutritional deficiencies and injuries to the joints. Obesity, which is reaching epidemic proportions in North America, is also a major contributing factor. Excess body weight puts additional strain on the joints and can lead to accelerated breakdown of cartilage. This is particularly problematic in the knees and hips.

Years of use, and especially abuse, can lead to wear and tear of the joint structure, specifically joint cartilage, resulting in osteoarthritis. Those engaged in certain sports, such as running, football, and basketball, and those whose daily work activities put strain on their joints, may be at increased risk of developing osteoarthritis earlier in life.

Key symptoms of osteoarthritis include:

- stiffness and swelling in one or more joints
- deep, aching pain in a joint
- pain associated with movement of a joint
- tenderness, warmth, or redness in afflicted joints
- fever, weight loss, or fatigue that accompanies joint pain

Since osteoarthritis frequently affects the spine, back pain is another common symptom. The diagnosis of osteoarthritis is based on a physical examination and a history of symptoms. X-rays are used to confirm diagnosis.

Keep in mind that osteoarthritis is quite different from rheumatoid arthritis. Actually, there are over 100 different types of arthritis. Rheumatoid arthritis is an autoimmune condition in which the immune system attacks the body's tissues as if they were foreign invaders. The symptoms of rheumatoid arthritis include inflammation of the membrane lining the joint or other internal organs, causing pain, stiffness, warmth, redness, and swelling. The disease is usually chronic, but can also be marked by flare-ups.

"Over time, chronic inflammation makes the joint lining thick and overgrown," according to *The Arthritis Cure,* by Jason Theodosakis, M.D. "This overgrown lining may then start to invade the cartilage, other joint-supporting tissues, and even the bone, weakening the entire joint structure." While SAMe has not been studied for rheumatoid arthritis, there is good evidence supporting its use in alleviating the pain of osteoarthritis.

Alleviating Osteoarthritis

Currently, there is no cure for osteoarthritis. The mainstream approach to the management of this disease centers upon decreasing pain and improving joint movement. Doctors will recommend certain exercises to keep the joints flexible and improve muscle strength. Devices such as knee braces may be used to protect the joint and provide support. Heat and cold therapy is sometimes used to provide temporary pain relief. Joint-replacement surgery is performed for severe cases when the joint damage is substantial and causes chronic pain.

The American College of Rheumatology (ACR) recommends weight loss and exercise for obese patients with osteoarthritis. This alone can help to relieve some of the pressure from the joints, thus reducing the pain, plus it benefits overall health. In a recent clinical study, researchers compared the effectiveness of a combination of long-term exercise and a healthy, calorie-restricted diet to the effects of exercise only, a calorie-restricted diet only, and a healthy lifestyle control group (given advice only but not put on exercise program or restricted diet) in a group of overweight patients with knee osteoarthritis. The results of their unique study were published in the May 2004 print issue of *Arthritis & Rheumatism.* It was found that patients who combined moderate exercise and a calorie-restricted diet had an average gain of 24 percent in their ability to perform daily activities, accompanied by a reduction in morning stiffness. This group also lost more weight—5.7 percent of total body weight, on average—than any other group.

The Perils of Prescription Drugs for Osteoarthritis

The most commonly prescribed class of drugs for managing the pain and inflammation of osteoarthritis is the nonsteroidal anti-inflammatory drugs (NSAIDs). These drugs work by decreasing the activity of an enzyme called cyclo-oxygenase, thereby inhibiting the formation of inflammatory chemicals known as prostaglandins. Examples of drugs in this class are ibuprofen, naproxen, flurbiprofen, diclofenac, indomethacin, and the new-generation drugs celecoxib (Celebrex®) and rofecoxib (Vioxx®).

While the NSAIDs are popularly prescribed, their use and benefits are hindered by numerous side effects and drug interactions. Many of the side effects are actually linked to the reduction of prostaglandin synthesis. Although prostaglandins are involved in the inflammatory response, they also have many beneficial effects in the body. They protect the stomach lining, promote clotting of the blood, regulate salt and fluid balance, and maintain blood flow to the kidneys when kidney function is reduced. Thus, by decreasing prostaglandins, NSAIDs can cause stomach irritation (nausea, pain, heartburn, and occasionally bleeding and perforation of the stomach or intestine), fluid retention, and reduced kidney function. Other side effects may include dizziness, skin rash, anemia, and decreased appetite. In rare cases they can also cause blood disorders, liver damage, and heart and kidney failure. These drugs should also be used cautiously by anyone taking anticoagulants, blood pressure medication, diuretics, and lithium.

Long-term NSAID use can also lead to the development of ulcers. It is estimated that prevalence of NSAID-induced gastric or duodenal ulcers varies between 14.6 percent and 43.9 percent (The *Journal of Rheumatology* 18[Supplement 28] [1991]:11–14). According to an article featured in *Pharmacoepidemiology and Drug Safety* (6[1996]:157-168), of the 1417 drug-related deaths reported in Canada from 1984 to 1994, nearly 12 percent were caused by anti-inflammatory and antirheumatic medications.

The "Warnings" section of the monograph for Motrin® (ibuprofen), as published in the *Compendium of Pharmaceuticals and Specialties* (Ottawa : Canadian Pharmacists Association, 2002), states that "ulceration, perforation and bleeding of the stomach, small intestine or large intestine, sometimes severe and occasionally fatal have been reported during therapy with nonsteroidal anti-inflammatory drugs (NSAIDs) including ibuprofen." It also states that the "Elderly, frail and debilitated patients appear to be at higher risk from a variety of adverse reactions from NSAIDs." Similar warnings appear in the monographs for other NSAIDs. Significantly, most individuals who take these drugs for management of osteoarthritis are elderly.

During my years of pharmacy practice, I have seen many individuals suffer from side effects and drug interactions while using NSAIDs. I often wondered if the side effects and risks of taking the drug were worse than the disease. For some patients, the answer was yes. I always cautioned patients who began taking these drugs about the potential side effects and what early warnings signs to look for—abdominal pain; black, tarry stools; and bleeding from the rectum are signs that there is bleeding in the gastrointestinal tract (stomach or intestines). Unfortunately, I knew of several patients who had experienced ulcers, bleeding, and other side effects with these NSAIDs. In some of these cases, the patient had taken the product for years before a problem developed.

Not only are the potential side effects serious and even life-threatening, studies have shown that NSAIDs block cartilage repair and speed up cartilage destruction (*The Lancet* ii[I] [1985]:1–13). In other words, the drugs can actually make osteoarthritis worse by causing further breakdown of cartilage in the joint.

Finally, NSAID usage has also been linked to nutrient deficiencies. For example, indomethacin can decrease the absorption of folic acid, vitamin C, and possibly calcium. It may also interfere with the actions of vitamin C. The newer generation NSAID, celecoxib (Celebrex®), can also deplete folic acid levels in the body. Folic acid deficiency is known to be harmful to DNA metabolism, causing abnormal cellular development.

Deficiency can also lead to anemia, cervical dysplasia, and elevated homocysteine (a newly recognized factor in heart disease). If levels are deficient during pregnancy, it can also lead to neural tube defects in the child. Iron levels may also be reduced in those taking NSAIDs over the long term.

Considering the many risks and concerns connected with NSAID usage, it is critical to consider other options for the management of osteoarthritis—safer and more natural approaches, such as SAMe.

SAMe and Osteoarthritis

You may be wondering what led researchers to make the jump from depression to osteoarthritis. It was chance, according to Geoffrey Cowley of *Newsweek* magazine. It appears that researchers stumbled upon this additional benefit when participants in a depression study reported that their osteoarthritis symptoms had also improved.

From a biochemical standpoint, this added benefit makes perfect sense because SAMe plays an important role in both cartilage formation and repair. Evidence suggests that SAMe directly stimulates the production of chondrocytes (cartilage cells). It has also been shown to increase the incorporation of sulfur into proteoglycans, the starting material for cartilage formation. As well, SAMe has been shown to have both anti-inflammatory and analgesic properties, although the mechanism by which it achieves these effects is not clear. It is known that SAMe does not work via the prostaglandin system like the NSAIDs do.

Supporting Research on Osteoarthritis

The benefits and value of SAMe in alleviating the pain of osteoarthritis were recently reviewed and reported by the U.S. Department of Health and Human Services, Agency for

Healthcare Research and Quality (AHRQ). Investigators reviewed ten studies that involved using SAMe to treat osteoarthritis. Some of these studies compared SAMe to a placebo and others compared it to standard NSAIDs. The investigators reported that ". . . SAMe has modest but significant benefit compared to placebo and no difference in efficacy between SAMe and NSAIDs." As with depression, SAMe was found to be more effective than a placebo and equally effective as the commonly prescribed prescription drugs.

Another review of clinical studies involving SAMe as an osteoarthritis treatment came to the same conclusion: "The intensity of therapeutic activity of SAMe against osteoarthritis is similar to that exerted by non-steroidal anti-inflammatory drugs (NSAIDs)." (*American Journal of Medicine* 83[5A] [1987]:60–65).

In addition, animal studies have shown that SAMe actually restores damaged cartilage and protects the stomach lining—just the opposite of what popular NSAIDs have been shown to do. As I mentioned, bleeding ulcers and joint cartilage destruction are two possible side effects of long-term NSAID usage.

Here are highlights of some clinical studies of the use of SAMe for treating osteoarthritis:

1. *SAMe vs. naproxen:* This double-blind, multicenter study evaluated the efficacy and tolerability of SAMe in comparison to a placebo and naproxen in the treatment of osteoarthritis of the hip, knee, spine, and hand. A total of 734 subjects, including 582 with hip or knee osteoarthritis, were enrolled. SAMe (given orally at a dose of 1200 mg daily) was shown to exert the same analgesic activity as naproxen (750 mg daily). Both drugs were more effective than a placebo. Tolerability of SAMe was significantly better than that of naproxen, both in terms of physicians' and patients' judgments and in terms of the number of patients with side effects. There was no difference between SAMe and a placebo in the number of side effects (Caruso 1987).

2. *SAMe vs. ibuprofen:* This double-blind, multicenter, randomized clinical trial compared the effects of ibuprofen to SAMe in 150 patients with knee and/or hip osteoarthritis. Both drugs were given orally 400 mg three times daily for thirty days. The authors concluded that "SAMe exhibited a slightly more marked activity than the reference drug in the management of the various painful manifestations of the joint disease. Minor side-effects developed in five patients of SAMe group, and in 16 patients of ibuprofen group. No dropouts occurred" (Marcolongo 1985).

3. *SAMe vs. piroxicam:* Forty-five patients completed this double-blind, randomized, twelve-week trial comparing 1200 mg of SAMe daily with 20 mg of piroxicam (another NSAID) daily. Both treatments proved effective in reducing total pain scores, but SAMe was slightly more effective. As well, patients treated with SAMe maintained clinical improvement longer than patients receiving the piroxicam (Maccagno et al. 1987).

4. *SAMe vs. ibuprofen*: In this double-blind study, thirty-six patients with osteoarthritis of the knee, hip, and/or spine were given 1200 mg of SAMe or 1200 mg of ibuprofen (a very commonly prescribed NSAID) for four weeks. SAMe performed equally as well as ibuprofen. The researchers assessed morning stiffness, pain at rest, pain on motion, crepitus, swelling, and limitation of motion of the affected joints before and after treatment. Symptom scores improved to the same extent in patients treated with SAMe or ibuprofen (Muller-Fassbender 1987).

5. The largest study to date on SAMe included over 20,000 osteoarthritis patients (Berger 1987). This two-month study evaluated the effects of a sliding dose of SAMe. Patients received 1200 mg for the first week, 800 mg the second week,

and then 400 mg from weeks three to eight. SAMe was given in divided doses on an empty stomach and no additional anti-inflammatory drugs or analgesics were used in the study. The results were as follows: very good or good, 71 percent; moderate results, 21 percent; and poor, 9 percent. SAMe was well tolerated by the individuals in most cases: good, 87 percent; moderate, 8 percent; and poor, 5 percent. Gastrointestinal upset was the most common side effect reported. A limitation of this study is that it did not include comparison with a placebo or another osteoarthritis drug (NSAID).

Patient Case 3: Osteoarthritis

DESCRIPTION

Fred, a seventy-seven-year-old male, was diagnosed with osteoarthritis of the back, hips, and knees in 1984. His condition had progressed to the point where he had been unable to walk for the past three years and could stand only for brief periods. Symptoms included pain, discomfort, and lack of mobility.

PREVIOUS TREATMENT

Over the previous ten years, Fred had been on various arthritis medications, including ibuprofen, indomethacin, and diclofenac. He noticed blood in his stool and was diagnosed with NSAID-induced gastric ulcer in 1998. His doctor ordered him to discontinue NSAID usage. One week later the pain in his knees and back became intolerable. He came to the pharmacy one day and asked me if there was anything that I could recommend that wouldn't hurt his stomach.

RECOMMENDATION

I suggested that Fred try SAMe for his osteoarthritis pain. He began taking 400 mg of SAMe daily and gradually built up to 1200 mg daily, increasing the dose at two-week intervals.

FOLLOW-UP

Within thirty days he noticed that his pain was subsiding, and two months later he noticed significant improvement in all joint areas. He was able to start his walking program again and had greater flexibility. He stated that "For the first time in almost three years, I am able to walk pain-free." Three months after discontinuing his diclofenac, his ulcer had healed and Fred was feeling better than he had in years.

Patient Case 4: Osteoarthritis

DESCRIPTION

Emma came to see me one day regarding the pain in her knees, elbows, and wrists. Her doctor had diagnosed it as osteoarthritis. When she was younger, Emma loved to run and play tennis. She had participated in many marathons and had even won several awards for her athletic ability. Now in her mid-sixties, she still enjoyed exercise and had recently taken up golf and power walking. Over time Emma was finding it difficult to get up from a squatting or sitting position and was experiencing aching pain in her wrists, elbows, and knees.

PREVIOUS TREATMENT

Since Emma had weak kidney function and was taking certain medications, she was not a candidate for NSAID therapy. Her doctor recommended that she talk to me about other options.

RECOMMENDATION

I recommended that Emma wear a wrist brace for support during the night and as much as possible during the day. I also suggested that she invest in a pair of walking shoes that would provide good cushioning and support. To help repair the underlying joint damage and alleviate pain, I suggested that she try 400 mg of SAMe twice daily.

FOLLOW-UP

Six weeks later, Emma came back to the pharmacy to thank me for my recommendations. She had found tremendous benefits with the SAMe and the other suggestions that I provided. Emma was able to increase her activity level to golf twice a week and daily power walks. She also commented that she felt better emotionally—her spirits were lifted and she had more energy. I shared with Emma the other side benefit of our natural superstar—as a mood elevator. She was surprised to learn that SAMe had positive rather than negative side effects.

In summary, considering the prevalence of osteoarthritis, the serious problems associated with NSAID usage, and the substantial evidence supporting the benefits of SAMe, the discovery of SAMe as an osteoarthritis treatment is a significant breakthrough.

Let's review the key points about using SAMe for osteoarthritis:

- SAMe plays an important role in cartilage formation and repair.
- It helps to alleviate the pain and inflammation of osteoarthritis.
- Clinical studies have found SAMe comparable in efficacy to commonly prescribed NSAIDs, but better tolerated.
- SAMe has international recognition as a therapeutic agent for osteoarthritis.
- SAMe has a strong safety record. While most osteoarthritis drugs damage the stomach lining, SAMe has been shown to actually protect the stomach lining.

As I discussed in the introduction, SAMe is involved in many important body functions. It is almost unbelievable that a safe, natural substance can be effective for so many different types of conditions. I have to admit that I was skeptical at first when

I heard about all the purported health benefits of SAMe. However, a thorough review of the scientific evidence, combined with an understanding of how SAMe works in the body, makes it far easier to accept the fact that this substance provides many different benefits.

For example, it becomes easy to understand why SAMe is so safe when you consider that it is actually manufactured in the human body to perform and assist with many different tasks. Supplementing with SAMe makes sense when you consider its myriad benefits and the fact that SAMe levels are depleted in certain individuals. Keep in mind, however, that not everything manufactured in the human body is safe and useful. Toxic free radicals occur as a result of many internal functions, as well as external influences (e.g., pollution, smoking, pesticides, and hormones). However, the human body has a team of internal controls and mechanisms to keep us healthy and take care of these damaging free radicals. SAMe is one of those internal team members working on our behalf.

Because of its involvement in many vital biochemical processes that affect human health, SAMe can benefit a wide range of conditions. While the evidence is strongest for depression and osteoarthritis, mounting research is supporting the use of SAMe for fibromyalgia, chronic fatigue syndrome, and liver disease. I will explore these areas in the following sections.

Fibromyalgia/Chronic

FIBROMYALGIA/CHRONIC FATIGUE SYNDROME

Fibromyalgia (FM) is a fairly new diagnosis. In fact, the classification criteria for diagnosing the illness has been available for only fifteen years. A key characteristic of FM is chronic pain in muscles and soft tissues surrounding joints. Physicians diagnose FM if eleven of eighteen identified tender points are painful to touch. These tender spots, called trigger points, exist in different spots throughout the body. The most commonly affected locations are on the occiput (nape of the neck), the neck itself, shoulders, trunk, lower back, and thighs. Other symptoms include sleep disturbance, depression, fatigue, abdominal pain, and swollen lymph nodes.

It is estimated that 3 to 6 million people are affected by this disorder in the United States, the vast majority of them women between twenty-five and forty-five.

Chronic fatigue syndrome (CFS) is a related syndrome, and can be just as vague and difficult to diagnose as fibromyalgia. While pain is the key symptom of FM, extreme fatigue is the primary symptom of CFS. Physicians diagnose CFS when there is severe, relapsing fatigue that cannot be explained or attributed to any other illness. In addition to fatigue, several of the following symptoms are also present with CFS: mild fever, sore throat, muscle weakness, generalized headache, forgetfulness, irritability, confusion, inability to concentrate, sleep disturbances, and depression. CFS is also most common among women ages twenty-five to forty-five. According to some reports, between 100 and 300 individuals per 100,000 have CFS.

Initially, the medical community considered FM and CFS to be psychological disorders, possibly due to hypochondria or neurosis. Today, however, the scientific community has recognized that these are very real and complex conditions, yet there is still a stigma associated with these conditions because the underlying cause has not yet been determined.

There are various psychological symptoms in both FM and CFS, but there is a wide range of other symptoms that these individuals experience. Some researchers have theorized that a virus or infections could trigger these diseases. It has also been suggested that these conditions may arise from environmental toxicity or trauma, but this is still speculation.

Present treatment for both of these conditions focuses on symptomatic relief—reducing pain, improving sleep, and maintaining function. No cure for either illness is currently known. Some of the commonly prescribed drugs for these conditions include antidepressants, muscle relaxants, anti-inflammatory drugs, and analgesics. In some patients, antidepressant therapy helps to improve sleep and well-being and reduce fatigue, but has no effect on the pain and trigger points. Unfortunately, many patients are left to struggle with a poor quality of life and an exhausting list of symptoms and problems associated with these conditions.

Supporting Research on Fibromyalgia

Since SAMe is known to address symptoms that are common to FM and CFS, such as joint pain and swelling, as well as depression, researchers felt that it may hold promise for the management of FM and CFS. As it turns out, SAMe is believed to be one of the most widely studied natural substances for FM that exists today—even though only been a few studies completed. The results of these studies have been very positive for FM sufferers. So far, there have been no clinical studies with SAMe for the treatment of CFS, but there have been a number of positive case reports.

With respect to FM, several studies have determined that people with this condition often have low serotonin levels in their blood. Serotonin is an important neurotransmitter (chemical messenger) that regulates mood and well-being. One of SAMe's mechanisms for alleviating depression is boosting levels of serotonin, which is believed to be the reason why SAMe is helpful for managing FM.

Clinical studies on SAMe for fibromyalgia have used both injectable and oral forms. Below are some highlights from a few of these studies:

1. *Department of Rheumatology, Frederiksberg Hospital, Copenhagen (Jacobson et al. 1991)*: In this double-blind trial, researchers gave forty-four patients diagnosed with primary

fibromyalgia either 800 mg of SAMe orally daily or a placebo, for six weeks. Improvements were seen for clinical disease activity, pain experienced during the last week, fatigue, morning stiffness, and mood in those treated with SAMe. There was no difference between groups in the tender point score, isokinetic muscle strength, mood as evaluated by the Beck Depression Inventory, and side effects. The authors concluded that "S-adenosylmethionine has some beneficial effects on primary fibromyalgia and could be an important option in the treatment hereof."

2. *Institute of Medical Pathology I, University of Pisa (Tavoni et al. 1987)*: This study compared the effect of 200 mg of SAMe (given intramuscularly) to a placebo in a double-blind crossover study of seventeen patients with primary fibromyalgia. Eleven of seventeen patients had a significant depressive state. The number of trigger points, plus painful anatomic sites, decreased after administration of SAMe, but not after placebo treatment. In addition, depression scores improved after SAMe administration, whereas they did not significantly change after placebo treatment. The researchers concluded that "SAMe treatment, by improving the depressive state and reducing the number of trigger points, seems to be an effective and safe therapy in the management of primary fibromyalgia."

3. *Department of Rheumatology, Frederiksberg Hospital, Copenhagen (Volkmann 1997)*: Thirty-four out-patients with fibromyalgia symptoms received 600 mg of SAMe intravenously or a placebo daily for ten days in a crossover trial. There was no significant difference in improvement in the tender points; however, there were some benefits in subjective perception of pain at rest, pain on movement, and overall well-being, and a slight improvement in fatigue, quality of

sleep, morning stiffness, and on the Fibromyalgia Impact Questionnaire for pain. A limitation of this study was its small sample size and very short duration (ten days).

SAMe's role in treating the emotional and physical aspects of FM is very promising. Considering the growing number of people struggling with these conditions and the limitations of prescription drug treatments, SAMe could fill an important therapeutic gap.

LIVER DISORDERS

Liver Disorders

Chronic and acute liver diseases affect millions of people every year. The most common types of liver disease are cirrhosis, hepatitis, and drug-induced liver damage. At present, very few therapeutic agents effectively alleviate the symptoms of these diseases. Because of the vital role the liver plays in our health, even minor liver problems can have far-reaching negative health effects in the body. In addition, cholestasis (i.e., obstruction of the bile duct resulting in diminished or halted bile flow) can become a serious and difficult-to-treat condition. Bile builds up and results in symptoms such as intense itching (pruritis) and a yellowing of the skin.

"One of the most common causes of bile-duct obstruction is the presence of gallstones," explains Dr. Murray in the *Encyclopedia of Nutritional Supplements*. "SAMe is apparently the perfect supplement to relieve a condition naturopathic physicians often refer to as 'sluggish liver.'"

Supporting Research on Liver Disorders

According to several clinical studies, SAMe shows promise as an effective new medicine to treat liver disease and support healthy liver function. Researchers have made these important connections between SAMe and liver function:

- SAMe levels are depleted in liver disease, and its replenishment through supplementation has been demonstrated in several studies.
- Due to its methylating properties, SAMe promotes the fluidity of liver lipid membranes. It works directly with the cells of the liver to improve function of cell receptors, enzymes, and cell transporters.
- It has been shown to improve liver health according to measures of standard liver and liver function tests.
- Due to its supportive role in detoxification, SAMe can protect against liver toxicity induced by drugs, alcohol, and other chemicals.
- SAMe increases hepatic glutathione levels in patients with both alcohol and non-alcoholic cirrhosis. Glutathione is an important antioxidant that has been shown to protect the liver (and many other organs) from oxidative stress and drug-induced liver toxicity. (I'll discuss the importance of glutathione further on in the anti-aging section.)
- Animal experiments suggest the possibility that it could be useful as a chemopreventive agent—to protect against liver tumors—through its apparent ability to inhibit the expression of some oncogene (cancer gene) functions.

Researchers in London conclude that "SAMe has established biochemical and biophysical effects, which in pilot studies ameliorate symptoms and biochemical parameters of cholestasis . . . abnormalities in liver function tests also improve."

Here are the two most significant findings featured in the scientific literature regarding the benefits of supplements of SAMe on liver health:

1. SAMe was shown to restore normal liver function in the presence of various chronic liver diseases, including alcoholic and non-alcoholic cirrhosis and estrogen-induced cholestasis.

2. It prevented and reversed liver toxicity caused by several drugs and chemicals, including alcohol, acetaminophen, steroids, and lead.

Specific to cholestasis, two important preliminary studies were conducted. The first involved thirty pregnant women in their last trimester diagnosed with obstructed bile flow to the liver. No adverse effects occurred with the mother or child during SAMe treatment. Even more significant, both subjective and objective signs of the condition were improved when compared to a placebo.

The other study involved 220 cholestatic patients who also had chronic liver disease. The study demonstrated that SAMe was more effective than a placebo, was very well tolerated, and "offers a new therapeutic modality for the symptomatic management of this syndrome," according to the researchers.

SAMe has even been studied for the most feared liver disease of all, liver cancer. SAMe supplementation had a significant protective effect against liver cancer in animals exposed to liver cancer–causing agents. "One of the greatest risks of chronic liver diseases, such as chronic hepatitis, is liver cancer," explains Dr. Murray. "Supplementation with SAMe is very much indicated in patients with these diseases in order to reduce the risk for liver cancer."

The *Evidence Report on SAMe*, prepared by the U.S. Department of Health and Human Services, Agency for Healthcare Research and Quality (AHRQ), reported the following:

- Compared to placebo, treatment with SAMe for cholestasis of pregnancy was associated with a large effect in decreasing pruritus and in decreasing bilirubin levels.
- Compared to a placebo for intrahepatic cholestasis, treatment with SAMe for pruritis was associated with a risk ratio of 0.45, meaning that patients treated with SAMe

were twice as likely as placebo-treated patients to have a reduction in pruritus.

Of course, more research is needed in this area before SAMe can be used as a primary treatment option for people with a weak liver or a challenging liver disorder. So far, however, preliminary results look promising. If they are confirmed, SAMe could prove to be an important therapy for liver health.

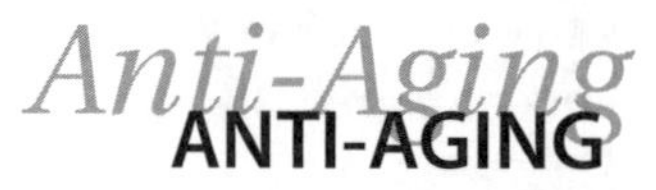

ANTI-AGING

We know that SAMe, as an active methyl donor, plays a vital role in many major body functions. The most significant activity is believed to occur in the brain. Earlier studies confirmed that oral SAMe does cross the blood-brain barrier. This means that after SAMe is taken, it travels to the brain and actually penetrates brain tissue. This is significant because many substances do not cross the blood-brain barrier and therefore do not reach the neurotransmitters located in the brain. In order for a substance to provide any benefit to brain function and positively affect mood, it must be able to influence neurotransmitters by crossing the blood-brain barrier.

For these reasons, SAMe may also be useful in treating other conditions of the central nervous system. It has been studied for treating dementia, which is a progressive failure in thought processes caused by brain damage or disease. Alzheimer's disease is a leading cause of dementia. By checking cerebrospinal fluid, Italian researcher Bottiglieri and colleagues discovered that SAMe levels were low in a group of patients with Alzheimer's dementia. An interesting earlier animal study by Japanese researchers demonstrated that SAMe improved recovery from brain disturbances.

Although preliminary, both of these studies indicate that SAMe may provide further neurological benefit. Clearly, one of the most distressing illnesses associated with aging is senile dementia. Perhaps studies will indicate that SAMe can help prevent this from occurring.

In addition to its neurological effects, SAMe also increases glutathione levels. This could prove to be the most important anti-aging benefit that SAMe provides.

All cells within the body contain glutathione, a powerful antioxidant. The highest concentrations of glutathione are found in the liver, lenses of the eyes, spleen, pancreas, and kidneys. According to Elson Haas, M.D., glutathione "is a key protector from potential damage by wastes and toxins and is effective in preventing aging."

Glutathione helps detoxify the system and plays a role in protecting cells from damage. In this sense, glutathione can help prevent a wide range of diseases associated with aging, including cancer, stroke, heart disease, and cataracts.

"Glutathione assumes a critical role in detoxification and defense against a variety of injurious agents by combining directly with these toxic substances to eventually form water-soluble compounds" that the body can then eliminate, states Dr. Murray.

Furthermore, glutathione can also directly disarm free radicals and enhance immune system activity. It transports important nutrients to immune system cells, such as lymphocytes, phagocytes, and macrophages.

Glutathione keeps red blood cells strong and helps protect all cells and membranes within the body. Obviously, this substance is important to our health. This is also a prime example of the powerful healing capabilities our bodies possess.

The relationship SAMe has to increased glutathione levels is a definite health benefit. Hopefully, further research will confirm the many health-promoting effects of this relationship.

New Areas of Research

NEW AREAS OF RESEARCH

Research on SAMe continues and exciting new areas are being explored. One aspect that is being investigated is SAMe's ability to lower lipids (cholesterol). There is a single study, apparently without follow-up, showing that SAMe might be an effective agent for lowering lipids in humans.

Another promising area is the use of SAMe to treat Parkinson's-associated depression. A small study conducted at Beth Israel Medical Center–Albert Einstein College of Medicine in New York found some positive results. This study examined the effects of SAMe on thirteen depressed patients with Parkinson's disease. All the patients had previously been treated with other antidepressant agents, with no significant benefit or with intolerable side effects. SAMe was administered in doses of 800–3600 mg per day for ten weeks. Eleven patients completed the study, and ten had at least a 50 percent improvement on the seventeen-point Hamilton Depression Scale. One patient did not improve and two patients dropped out because of increased anxiety. Side effects were mild and transient. Although this study was small, the authors concluded that "SAM is well tolerated and may be a safe and effective alternative to the antidepressant agents currently used in patients with Parkinson's disease."

SAMe deficiencies have also been found in individuals who have nerve damage from HIV/AIDS, multiple sclerosis, or spinal cord degeneration. SAMe is an important ingredient in reactions used to make a substance that holds myelin, the coating on nerve fibers, together. It is believed that supplemental SAMe may delay or prevent the spinal cord deterioration (myelopathy) that often accompanies infection with HIV. A study is currently enrolling patients with HIV to evaluate methionine's effectiveness in treating myelopathy (Szalavitz 1999).

Other areas of promise for SAMe include the management of adult attention deficit hyperactivity disorder (ADHD). A recent study found SAMe helpful in relieving the symptoms of ADHD. Individuals with migraine headaches have responded favorably to taking 200–400 mg of SAMe twice daily. This was reported in a study that evaluated the benefits of SAMe for intrahepatic cholestasis. More research is needed before SAMe can be recommended for these conditions.

SUPPLEMENTING WITH SAMe

Since it is virtually impossible to get therapeutic amounts of SAMe from the diet, those desiring the health benefits discussed in this booklet should consider a SAMe supplement.

As well, certain individuals who have a deficiency or reduced production of SAMe should consider supplements, including the elderly and those with:

- deficiency of methionine, vitamin B12, or folic acid, which can result from poor diet or use of prescription drugs that deplete these nutrients (estrogens, anticonvulsants, antidepressants, and certain blood pressure medications)
- depression
- osteoarthritis
- liver disease

In many European countries SAMe is actually classified and prescribed as a drug. In North America, however, SAMe is sold as a dietary supplement and can be found in health food stores and pharmacies. Look for the name Isoactive High Isomer SAMe to be sure you are getting the natural form of SAMe. I will discuss the reason for this later on.

Adverse Reactions

ADVERSE REACTIONS

SAMe is very safe and well tolerated. There have not been any reports of serious adverse events in those taking SAMe in doses up to 1600 mg per day over long periods. Reported side effects include mild gastrointestinal upset (nausea, diarrhea, and flatulence), anxiety, hyperactive muscle movement, insomnia, and hypomania. When these side effects occur, they often diminish with time or are resolved with lower doses or cessation of use. There are no documented cases of allergies to SAMe.

Interactions

INTERACTIONS

There are no reported adverse interactions with SAMe and other drugs, dietary supplements, or foods. However the possibility exists with the following drugs:

- *Standard antidepressants*: Do not take SAMe except on a physician's advice.
- *Medications for manic-depressive disease*: Do not take SAMe except on a physician's advice.
- *Levodopa for Parkinson's disease*: This is a positive interaction—SAMe might help the Parkinson's drug to work better.

Dosage Guidelines

DOSAGE GUIDELINES AND STORAGE

SAMe is most frequently available in 400 and 800 mg tablets. The usual oral dose for use in depression has been in the range of 400–1600 mg daily in divided doses. For liver problems, usual doses reported are up to 1600 mg daily in divided doses. For joint health, the daily dose is typically 400–1200 mg in divided doses. SAMe should always be taken on an empty stomach—one hour before meals or two hours after meals. Once a positive response has been achieved, it may be possible to reduce the dosage. Allow two weeks for the optimum therapeutic effect.

It is recommended to take SAMe along with supplements of B6, B12, folic acid, and possibly trimethylglycine (particularly in those with elevated homocysteine levels). These other nutrients help metabolize homocysteine, which, at elevated levels, may increase the risk of cardiovascular disease and some other disorders. SAMe has not been found to elevate homocysteine levels, yet the possibility exists. Some manufacturers combine SAMe with these nutrients. If your formula does not, then choose a good-quality multivitamin or B-complex that does.

SAMe is highly unstable at temperatures above 32°F (0°C). Since the 1970s, certain salts of SAMe have become available that are stable at higher temperatures. These forms, which are clearly more desirable, include S-adenosylmethionine tosylate. Even this temperature-stable form must be kept very dry since moisture can cause hydrolysis. Stable, enteric-coated tablets are recommended.

BUYER BE WISE

Buyer Be Wise

Consumers are becoming sophisticated shoppers. Word of mouth and testimonials are not enough. Here are the two most important components necessary to create a supplement "superstar": (1) scientific evidence published in peer-reviewed medical journals in the form of clinical research that proves its effectiveness and (2) a solid safety record with a clear indication of low toxicity and little risk. Certainly, SAMe meets these criteria and deserves its current stardom.

Natural Isoactive Versus

NATURAL ISOACTIVE VERSUS SYNTHETIC SAMe

Since SAMe is regulated as a dietary supplement in North America, there are a few things to keep in mind when purchasing a SAMe supplement. The following guidelines can help you purchase the highest-quality SAMe product:

1. Choose an enteric-coated tablet. If the product is not enteric coated, it will degrade rapidly. If the product has a strong egg-like odor, it could be degrading.
2. The label must indicate the total milligram amount of SAMe in the total salt form (i.e., tosylate or toluene disulfonate), and then list the milligram amount or percentage of the active ingredient. Look for a product that has a detailed, descriptive label. The more information provided, the better.
3. Choose a product from a reputable manufacturer with a history of supplying quality supplements.
4. Don't automatically buy the cheapest brand—you may be wasting your money on an inferior product that will not deliver results.
5. Look for natural "*Isoactive High Isomer SAMe.*" While synthetic (generic) SAMe is available on the market at a fraction of the price of the natural form, it does not deliver the same benefits. **Only the natural form of SAMe, sold as Isoactive High Isomer SAMe, provides a high ratio of the active SS Isomer of SAMe**—this isomer is responsible for the health benefits. As well, only the natural form of SAMe has been clinically tested. SAMe is an example of a case where the synthetic form is not equal to the natural form. The bottom line is that the cheaper, generic product will probably provide no benefit, or you'll have to take a much higher quantity, which will cost you more in the long run.

Conclusion

CONCLUSION

While the health benefits of SAMe are numerous and wide ranging, it is not a cure-all. Substantial evidence exists to support the use of SAMe for the following conditions: depression, osteoarthritis, fibromyalgia, and liver disorders. SAMe may also benefit people with chronic fatigue syndrome, migraine headaches, dementia, and HIV/AIDS. More research is needed in these areas before I can confidently recommend SAMe for these conditions, but it looks promising.

As a pharmacist, I strongly believe in the value of quality nutritional supplements such as Isoactive SAMe. Its strong safety profile and solid clinical research make it a true superstar in the supplement industry. I have recommended this product for many of my patients who were struggling with depression, osteoarthritis, fibromyalgia, and liver disease and the results have been tremendous. SAMe is a remarkable product that can help support overall health and reduce the symptoms of these chronic diseases.

Whether you are dealing with a certain illness discussed in this booklet, or you are interested in prevention, keep in mind that lifestyle choices play a critical role in overall health and wellness. A healthy diet, regular exercise, not smoking, stress management, adequate sleep, and a positive attitude are all lifestyle choices that help to determine our state of health or disease. These are factors that we have control over and can use to our advantage to reduce our risk of disease.

References

REFERENCES

Barcelo, H.A., J.C. Wiemeyer, C.L. Sagasta, M. Maclas, and J.C. Barreira. 1987. “Effect of S-adenosylmethionine on Experimental Osteoarthritis in Rabbits.” *American Journal of Medicine* 83(5A):55–59.

Bell, K.M., S.G. Potkin, D. Carreon, and L. Plon. 1994. “S-adenosylmethionine Blood Levels in Major Depression: Changes with Drug Treatment.” *Acta neurologica Scandinavica Supplementum* 154:15–18.

Berger, R., and H. Nowak. 1987. “A New Medical Approach to the Treatment of Osteoarthritis: Report of an Open Phase IV Study with Ademetionine.” *American Journal of Medicine* 83(5A): 84–88.

Berlanga, C., H.A. Ortega-Soto, M. Ontiveros, and H. Senties. 1992. “Efficacy of S-adenosyl-methionine in Speeding the Onset of Action of Imipramine.” *Psychiatry Research* 44(3):257–262.

Bottiglieri, T., P. Godfrey, T. Flynn, M.W. Carney, B.K. Toone, and E.H. Reynolds. 1990. "Cerebrospinal Fluid S-adenosyl-methionine in Depression and Dementia: Effects of Treatment with Parenteral and Oral S-adenosylmethionine." *Journal of Neurology, Neurosurgery, and Psychiatry* 53(12):1096–1098.

Bottiglieri, T., K. Hyland, and E.H. Reynolds. 1994. "The Clinical Potential of Ademethionine (S-adenosylmethionine) in Neurological Disorders." *Drugs* 48(2):137–152.

Bressa, G.M. 1994. "S-adenosyl-l-methionine (SAMe) as Antidepressant: Meta-analysis of Clinical Studies." *Acta neurologica Scandinavica Supplementum* 154:7–14.

Brooks, P.M., and R.O. Day. 1991. "Nonsteroidal Antiinflammatory Drugs: Differences and Similarities." *New England Journal of Medicine* 324(24):1716–1725.

Brown, R. 1999. Columbia University, personal interview, August 25.

Canadian Pharmacists Association. 2002. *Compendium of Pharmaceuticals and Specialties.* Ottawa: Canadian Pharmacists Association.

Carney, M.W., B.K. Toone, and E.H. Reynolds. "S-adenosyl-methionine and Affective Disorder." *American Journal of Medicine* 83(5A):104–106.

Caruso, I., and V. Pietrogrande. 1987. "Italian Double-Blind Multi-center Study Comparing S-adenosylmethionine, Naproxen, and Placebo in the Treatment of Degenerative Joint Disease." *American Journal of Medicine* 83(5A):66–71.

Cooney, C.A., C.K. Wise, L.A. Poirler, and S.F. Ali. 1998. "Methamphetamine Treatment Affects Blood and Liver S-adenosylmethionine (SAM) in Mice: Correlation with Dopamine Depletion in the Striatum." *Annals of the New York Academy of Sciences* 844:191–200.

Di Padova, C. 1987. "S-adenosylmethionine in the Treatment of Osteoarthritis: Review of Clinical Studies." *American Journal of Medicine* 83(5A):60–65.

Frezza, M., G. Centini, G. Cammareri, C. Le Grazie, and C. Di Padova. 1990. "S-adenosylmethionine for the Treatment of Intrahepatic Cholestasis of Pregnancy: Results of a Controlled Clinical Trial." *Hepatogastroenterology* 37(Supplement 2):122–125.

Frezza, M., C. Surrenti, G. Manzillo, F. Fiaccadori, M. Bortolini, and C. Di Padova. 1990. "Oral S-adenosylmethionine in the Symptomatic Treatment of Intrahepatic Cholestasis: A Double-Blind, Placebo-Controlled Study." *Gastroenterology* 99(l):211–215.

Friedel, H.A., K.L. Goa, and P. Benfield. 1989. "S-adenosyl-L-methionine: A Review of Its Pharmacological Properties and Therapeutic Potential in Liver Dysfunction and Affective Disorders in Relation to Its Physiological Role in Cell Metabolism." *Drugs* 38(3):389–416.

Geis, G.S., H. Stead, C.B. Wallermark et al. 1991. "Prevalence of Mucosal Lesions in the Stomach and Duodenum Due to Chronic Use of NSAIDs in Patients with Rheumatoid Arthritis or Osteoarthritis and Interim Report on Prevention by Misoprostol of Diclofenac Associated Lesions." *The Journal of Rheumatology* 18(Supplement 28):11–14.

Glorioso, S., S. Todesco, A. Mazzi et al. 1985. "Double-Blind Multicentre Study of the Activity of S-adenosylmethionine in Hip and Knee Osteoarthritis." *International Journal of Clinical Pharmacology Research* 5(1):39–49.

Goodnick, P.J., and R. Sandoval. 1993. "Psychotropic Treatment of Chronic Fatigue and Related Disorders." *Clinical Psychiatry* 54(l):13–20.

Gutierrez, S., I. Palacios, O. Sanchez-Pernaute, P. Hernandez, J. Moreno, J. Egido, and G. Herrera-Beaumont. 1997. "SAMe Restores the Changes in the Proliferation and in the Synthesis of Fibronectin and Proteoglycans Induced by Tumour Necrosis Factor Alpha in Cultured Rabbit Synovial cells." *British Journal of Rheumatology* 36(l):27–31.

Hardy, M., I. Coulter, S.C. Morton, et al. 2002. "S-Adenosyl-L-Methionine for Treatment of Depression, Osteoarthritis, and Liver Disease." Evidence Report, Technology Assessment Number 64. Prepared by Southern California Evidence-based Practice Center under Contract No. 290-97-001. AHRQ Publication No. 02-E034. Rockville: Agency for Healthcare Research and Quality.

Harmand, M.F., J. Vilamitjana, E. Maloche, R. Duphil, and D. Ducassou. 1987. "Effects of Sadenosylmethionine on Human Articular Chondrocyte Differentiation: An in vitro Study." *American Journal of Medicine* 83(5A):48–54.

Jacobsen, S., B. Danneskiold-Samsoe, and R.B. Anderson. 1991. "Oral S-adenosylmethionine in Primary Fibromyalgia: Double-Blind Clinical Evaluation." *Scandinavian Journal of Rheumatology* 20(4):294–302.

Janicak, P.G., J. Lipinski, J.M. Davis, E. Altmann, and R.P. Sharma. 1989. "Parenteral S-adenosylmethionine (SAMe) in Depression: Literature Review and Preliminary Data." *Psychopharmacology Bulletin* 25(2):238–242.

Kalbhen, D.A., and G. Jansen. 1990. "Pharmacologic Studies on the Antidegenerative Effect of Ademetionine in Experimental Arthritis in Animals." *Arzneimittelforschung* 40(9):1017–1021.

Laudanno, O.M. 1987. "Cytoprotective Effect of S-adenosylmethionine Compared with That of Misoprostal against Ethano-, Aspirin-, and Stress-Induced Gastric Damage." *American Journal of Medicine* 83(5A):43–47.

Linde, K., G. Ramirez, C.D. Mulrow, A. Pauls, W. Weidenhammer, and D. Melchart. 1996. "St. John's Wort for Depression: An Overview and Meta-analysis of Randomized Clinical Trials." *British Medical Journal* 313(7052):253–258.

Maccogno, A., E.E. Di Giorgio, O.L. Caston, and C.L. Sagasta. 1987. "Double-Blind Controlled Clinical Trial of Oral S-adenosylmethionine versus Piroxicam in Knee Osteoarthritis." *American Journal of Medicine* 83(5A):72–77.

Marcolongo N., N. Giordano, B. Colombo, et al. 1985. "Double-blind multicentre study of the activity of S-adenosylmethionine in hip and knee osteoarthritis." *Current Therapeutic Research* 37(1): 82–94.

Messier, S.P., R.F. Loeser, G.D. Miller et al. 2004. "Exercise and Dietary Weight Loss in Overweight and Obese Older Adults with Knee Osteoarthritis: The Arthritis, Diet, and Activity Promotion Trial." *Arthritis & Rheumatism* 50(5):1501–1510.

Muller-Fassbender, H. 1987. "Double-Blind Clinical Trial of S-adenosylmethionine versus Ibuprofen in the Treatment of Osteoarthritis." *American Journal of Medicine* 83(5A):81–83.

Murray, G., and R. Mayes. 1993. *Harpers Biochemistry*, 24th ed. Stamford: Appleton and Lang.

Murray, M. 1996. *Encyclopedia of Nutritional Supplements*. Rocklin: Prima Publishing.

Osman, E., J.S. Owen, and A.K. Burroughs. 1993. "Review Article: S-adenosyl-L-methionine: A New Therapeutic Agent in Liver Disease?" *Alimentary Pharmacology & Therapeutics* 7(l):21–28.

Parikh, S.V., and R.W. Lam. 2001. "Clinical Guidelines for the Treatment of Depressive Disorders. I. Definitions, Prevalence, and Health Burden." *Canadian Journal of Psychiatry* 46 (Supplement 1):13S–20S.

Peet, M. 1994. "Induction of Mania with Selective Serotonin Re-uptake Inhibitors and Tricyclic Antidepressants." *British Journal of Psychiatry* 164(4):549–550.

Reynolds, E.H., M.W. Carney, and B.K. Toone. 1984. "Methylation and Mood." *The Lancet* 4(8396):196–198.

Rosenbaum, J.F., M. Fava, W.E. Falk, M.H. Pollack, L.S. Cohen, B.M. Cohen, and G.S. Zubenko. 1990. "The Antidepressant Potential of Oral S-adenosyl-l-methionine." *Acta psychiatrica Scandinavica* 81(5):432–436.

Salmaggi, P., G.M. Bressa, G. Nicchia, M. Coniglio, P. La Greca, and C. Le Grazie. 1993. "Double-Blind, Placebo-Controlled

Study of S-adenosyl-L-methionine in Depressed Post-menopausal Women." *Psychotherapy and Psychosomatics* 59(l):34–40.

Stephens, T., and N. Joubert. 2001. "The Economic Burden of Mental Health Problems in Canada." *Chronic Diseases in Canada* 22(1):18–23.

Stramentinoli, G. 1987. "Pharmacologic Aspects of S-adenosylmethionine: Pharmacokinetics and Pharmaco-dynamics." *American Journal of Medicine* 83(5A):35–42.

Szalavitz, M. 1999. "SAMe as It Ever Was?" *Notes from the Underground* Spring (39):14–15.

Takahashi, J., H. Nishino, and T. Ono. 1986. "Effect of S-adenosyl-L-methionine on Disturbances in Hand Movement and Delayed Response Tasks after Lesion of Motor or Prefrontal Cortex in the Monkey." *Nippon Yakurigaku Zasshi* 87(5):507–519.

Tavoni, A., G. Jeracitano, and G. Cirigliano. 1998. "Evaluation of S-adenosylmethionine in Secondary Fibromyalgia: A Double-Blind Study." *Clinical and Experimental Rheumatology* 16(1):106–107.

Tavoni, A., C. Vitali, S. Bombardieri et al. 1987. "Evaluation of S-adenosylmethionine in Primary Fibromyalgia: A Double-Blind Crossover Study." *American Journal of Medicine* 83(Supplement 5A):107–110.

Theodosakis, J., B. Adderly, and B. Fox. 1997. *The Arthritis Cure.* New York: St. Martin's Press.

Thomas, C.L., ed. 1997. *Taber's Cyclopedic Medical Dictionary,* 18th ed. Philadelphia: E.A. Davis Co.

Thomson Healthcare Inc. 2004. PDRhealth Web site, S-Adenosyl-L-Methionine. <http://www.pdrhealth.com/drug_info/nmdrugprofiles/nutsupdrugs/sad_0231.shtml> Accessed June.

Tsuji, M., K. Kodama, and K. Oguchi. 1990. "Protective Effect of S-adenosyl-L-methionine against CC 14-Induced Hepatotoxicity in Cultured Hepatocytes." *Japanese Journal of Pharmacology* 52(2):209–214.

Vahora, S.A., and P. Malek-Ahmadi. 1988. "S-adenosylmethionine in the Treatment of Depression." *Neuroscience and Biobehavioral reviews* 12(2):139–141.

Volkmann, H., J. Norregaard, S. Jacobsen et al. 1997. "Double-Blind, Placebo-Controlled Cross-over Study of Intravenous S-adenosyl-L-methionine in Patients with Fibromyalgia." *Scandinavian Journal of Rheumatology* 26(3):206–211.